Sabrine Mejdoub Fehri

Chest CT and COVID-19

Sabrine Mejdoub Fehri

Chest CT and COVID-19

From diagnosis to care

ScienciaScripts

Imprint
Any brand names and product names mentioned in this book are subject to trademark, brand or patent protection and are trademarks or registered trademarks of their respective holders. The use of brand names, product names, common names, trade names, product descriptions etc. even without a particular marking in this work is in no way to be construed to mean that such names may be regarded as unrestricted in respect of trademark and brand protection legislation and could thus be used by anyone.

Cover image: www.ingimage.com

This book is a translation from the original published under ISBN 978-620-3-43461-3.

Publisher:
Sciencia Scripts
is a trademark of
Dodo Books Indian Ocean Ltd. and OmniScriptum S.R.L publishing group

120 High Road, East Finchley, London, N2 9ED, United Kingdom
Str. Armeneasca 28/1, office 1, Chisinau MD-2012, Republic of Moldova, Europe
Managing Directors: Ieva Konstantinova, Victoria Ursu
info@omniscriptum.com

Printed at: see last page
ISBN: 978-620-8-53751-7

TABLE OF CONTENTS

INTRODUCTION

At the end of December 2019, a series of cases of viral pneumonia caused by a new coronavirus appeared in Wuhan, China, and rapidly spread to all continents. This coronavirus, identified in airway samples, has been named SARS-CoV-2 for Severe Acute Respiratory Syndrome CoronaVirus-2 by the ICTV (International Committee on Taxonomy of Viruses) [1]. The disease it causes has been named COVID-19 for Coronavirus Disease 2019 by the WHO. SARS-CoV-2 belongs to the Coronaviridae family, like SARS-CoV and MERS-CoV, which were responsible for large-scale epidemics in 2003 and 2012 respectively [1]. The epidemic became an "international health emergency" at the end of January 2020 [2,3]. The most typical clinical presentation of COVID-19 is a febrile respiratory infection with dry cough, acute dyspnoea and myalgias. Approximately 15-20% of cases are severe and 2-3% are fatal [3-5]. It is essential to diagnose this disease as early as possible in order to isolate infected individuals and limit the spread of the epidemic. The reference diagnostic method is laboratory testing for viral RNA using RT-PCR (reverse transcriptase polymerase chain reaction) on nasopharyngeal swabs. While the specificity of the viral test is excellent, its sensitivity is imperfect (60-

70%) because it depends on the quality of the sample and the rate of viral replication in the upper respiratory tract [6-8]. Chest CT is an alternative, particularly for patients in respiratory distress whose treatment should not be delayed. For this reason, we conducted this study to determine the role of chest CT in the diagnosis and management of patients with COVID-19 infection.

PATIENTS AND METHODS

1. Type of study :

This is a retrospective and descriptive study including 251 patients hospitalised in the COVID-19 isolation unit at the University Hospital of Gabès, during the period from January to March 2021, 248 of whom had an initial thoracic CT scan.

2. Study population :

2.1. Inclusion criteria :

- Patients with SARS-CoV-2 infection confirmed by RT- PCR and radiological signs of COVID-19 pneumonia on chest scan

- Or the patients who had a thoracic scan with the presence of typical signs COVID-19 .

- Patients hospitalised in isolation unit COVID-19

➢ Lung involvement suggestive of SARS-CoV-2 infection on chest CT, according to the Société Française de Radiologie (SFR) , European Society of Radiology and the North American Society of

Radiology (RSNA) is characterised by a peripheral and bilateral ground-glass and/or multifocal ground-glass appearance with a rounded morphology with or without consolidation or visible intralobular lines ("crazypaving") and features of organised pneumonia, including the inverted halo sign. A posterior predominance of distribution has been reported in COVID-19 patients and was almost uniformly observed in typical cases.

- The extent of the anomalies is defined as: minimal (<10%), moderate (11-25%), significant (26-50%), severe (51-75%) and critical (>75 %).

2.2.Non-inclusion criteria :

- Patients who have not had a chest CT scan.

- The patients COVID -19 non hospitalised at the isolation unit COVID-19

3. Data collection :

We collected the following data from the records of patients admitted to the COVID-19 isolation unit, using individual computerised forms:

- Epidemiological characteristics (age, sex, smoking status, comorbidities).

- Characteristics COVID-19 infection

- Contage by SARS-CoV-2

- Diagnostic delay: this is the time between the onset of symptoms and the diagnosis. and consultation - Functional signs

- Diagnostic means

- Signs on clinical examination

- Biological data - Electrocardiogram

- Chest CT scan data

- Thoracic scanner technique

- Type and extent of radiological abnormalities

- Therapeutic management

- Ventilatory assistance

- Systemic corticosteroid therapy

- Antibiotic therapy

- Anti-coagulant

- Vitamin therapy - Evolution

4. Statistical analysis :

The data were entered using Microsoft Excel® and analysed using SPSS® version 20. For qualitative variables, we calculated simple frequencies and relative frequencies (percentages). For quantitative variables, we calculated averages and medians and determined the extreme values and standard deviation.

RESULTS

During the study period, 251 patients were admitted to the COVID-19 isolation unit, 248 of whom (98.8%) had a chest CT scan on admission.

1. General characteristics of the study population :

1.1. Age :

In our population, average age was 65 (18-100 years).

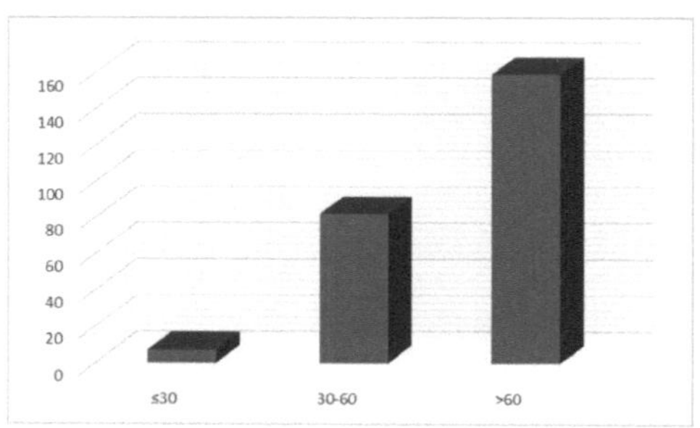

Figure 1: Breakdown by age group

1.2. sex :

In our series, 139 patients were male, i.e. 56% of cases.

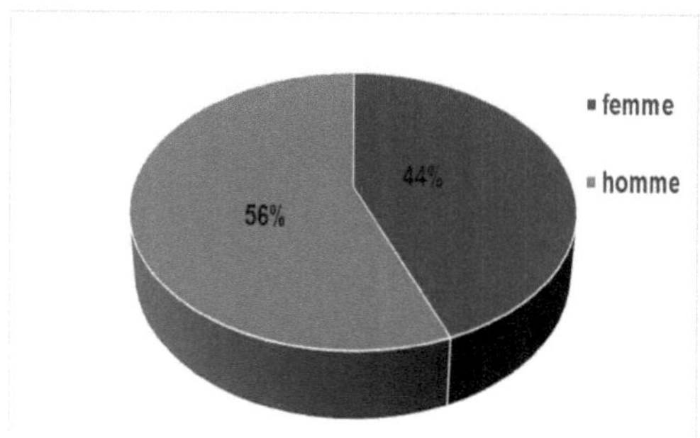

Figure 2: Breakdown by gender

1.3. Smoking status :

Twenty-five patients (10%) were smokers (of any type). For patients who used cigarettes, the average consumption 40 pack-years (p.a.) (from 5 to 100 p.a.).

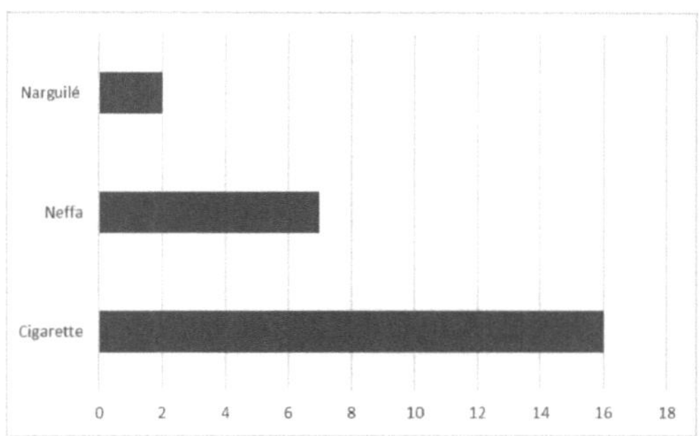

Figure 3: Distribution by type of tobacco intoxication

1.4. Comorbidities:

1.4.1. Respiratory history :

Respiratory history was noted in 11 cases (4.4%). (Table I)

1.4.2. Non-respiratory history :

A history of non-respiratory pathology was noted in 187 patients, i.e. 75.4% of cases. Ninety-one (48.6%) were hypertensive. Diabetes was noted in 81 patients (43.3%). (Table I)

Table I: Patients' medical history

Medical history Number Percentage

History	Asthma	5	2,6
respiratory	Bronchopneumopathy	3	1,6
	chronic obstructive		
	Pulmonary fibrosis	3	1,6
	Hypertension	91	48.6
	Diabetes	81	43.3
	extra-breathing Pathology cardiovascular	39	20.8
Accident vascular 11 5,8 brain			
Renal insufficiency	11	5,8	
Hypothyroidism	7	3,7	

2. Characteristics COVID infection- 19

2.1. Contage by SARS- COV2

Contact with a positive subject was found in 30 patients (12%).

2.2. Delay diagnosis

The diagnostic delay was 7 days (1-21 days).

2.3. Signs functional

Functional signs were dominated by dyspnoea (83.4%), cough (65.3%) and asthenia (47.1%). (Table II)

Table II: Functional signs

Functional signs	Number of patients	Percentage (%)
Dyspnoea	207	83
Cough	162	65
Asthenia	117	47
Fever	79	32
Headaches	71	29
Transit problems	62	25
Anosmia	16	6
Agueusia	14	5

2.4. Diagnostic means :

The diagnosis of SARS-COV2 infection was based on chest CT scans (in 119 patients: 48%) pending the results of RT-PCR, which was positive in 100 patients (84%). Only 112 patients (45%) were diagnosed on the basis of chest CT. And by chest CT combined with a positive rapid antigen test in 17 patients (7%).

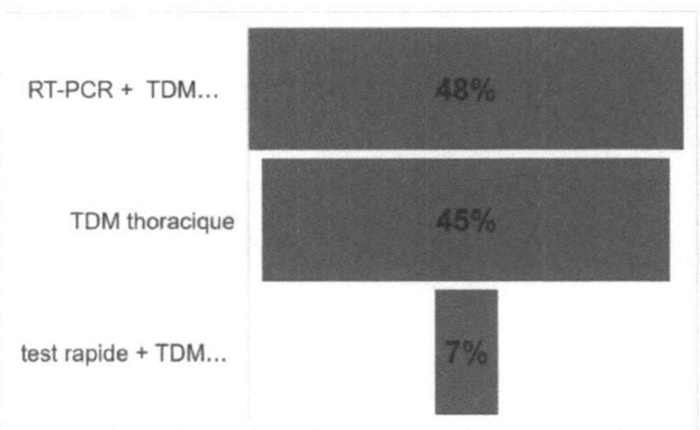

Figure 4: Breakdown by means of confirmation of SARS-CoV-2 infection

2.5. Clinical signs :

Fever was observed in 27 patients, with a mean temperature of 38.6° (37°-40°).Signs of acute respiratory failure were noted in 89% of patients, with signs of respiratory struggle, a mean respiratory rate of

28 c/min (20- 45 c/min) and a mean arterial oxygen saturation on room air of 79% (40%-88%).Lung auscultation revealed crackling rales in 171 patients (68%), snoring rales in 9 patients (3.6%) and sibilant rales in 5 patients (2%). Cardiovascular examination revealed tachycardia (HR>100 b/min) in 78% of patients and a mean blood pressure of 130/80 mmHg (100/50- 200/90 mmHg). Cardiac auscultation revealed an irregular rhythm in 2% of patients. Consciousness was preserved in the majority of patients. Only three patients (1%) had an altered neurological state with a glasgow score of S7.

2.6. Biological data

In the haematological tests, we noted leukopenia in 6.3% of cases, normal leukocytosis in 59.33% of cases and hyperleukocytosis in 34.36% of cases.Lymphopenia was noted in 47.3% of patients. Neutropenia was found in 6.6% of patients. Anaemia in women was around 20% and in men around 20.33%.We noted thrombocytosis in 6.6% of patients and thrombocytopenia in 16.6%. The mean CRP was 124mg/l (0-372 mg/l). D-dimer assays were requested in 229 patients, and were positive (>500ng/ml) in 24 patients with a mean level of 2239ng/ml (165- 10000ng/ml).

2.7. Electrocardiogram :

The ECG showed sinus tachycardia in 35% of patients, atrial fibrillation tachyarrhythmia in 2% and sinoatrial block in one case.

3. Chest CT scan data:

3.1. Chest CT technique :

Chest CT scans without injection of iodinated contrast were performed in 198 patients (80%) (Fig 5).

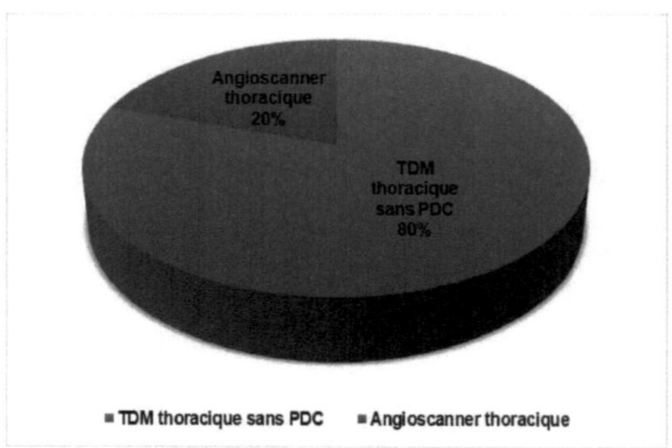

Figure 5:Breakdown by thoracic CT technique

3.2. Radiological abnormalities :

Types radiological anomalies (Table III)

An appearance suggestive of COVID-19 pneumonia was found in 227 cases (92%).Atypical COVID-19 pneumonia was found in 21 cases (8%). Abnormalities associated with the typical pulmonary involvement of COVID-19 were observed in 15% of patients. These included pulmonary embolism in 8% of cases and pleural effusion in 8%.

Table III:Types of abnormalities seen on chest CT scan

Types anomalies	Number of patients	Percentage (%)
Frosted glass	220	88
Condensations	45	18
Crazypaving	86	35
Perimeter thickening bronchovascular	15	6
Fine cross-linking	41	17
Pulmonary embolism	19	8
Pleural effusion	20	8

Chest CT revealed other abnormalities in 54 patients. cases (22%) (Table IV)

Table IV: Radiological abnormalities discovered by chance

Type fault	Number	percentage (%)
Adrenal adenoma	4	7 ,4
Centrosomatic vertebral angioma	3	5,5
Calcificationsvascula(aorta /coronary/ mitral valve)	3	5,5
Kidney stones	6	11
Cardiomegaly	5	9
Bronchial dilatation	5	9
Pericardial effusion	6	11
Hamartochondroma	1	1,8
Floating thrombus of the aorta	2	3 ,7
Pneumothorax	1	1,8
Emphysema	3	5,5
Anterior mediastinal mass	1	1,8
Spiculated pulmonary nodule	2	3,7
Mesenteric ischaemia	1	1,8
Vesicular lithiasis	3	5,5
PID	3	5,5
Kidney cyst	4	7,4
Thyroid nodule	4	7,4
Hiatus hernia	4	7,4

Topography of lesions :

Involvement was predominantly subpleural in 106 cases (43%), posterior in 87 cases (35%) and mixed in 108 cases.

- **Extent of pulmonary involvement :**

Bilateral involvement was reported in 217 cases (88%).

Involvement was severe, with >50% involvement in 127 cases (51%).

Table V: Degree of lung involvement

Degree damage	<10 %	10-25 %	25 - 50%	50-75	>75 %
Number of patients	4	27	90	87	40
Percentage (%)	1,6	10,8	36,3	35,1	16,2

4. Therapeutic management

4.1. Ventilatory assistance :

Oxygen therapy using a high concentration mask with a medium flow rate of 10 L/min was indicated in all patients. Non-invasive ventilation was indicated in 23% of patients. Mechanical ventilation was required in 3% of patients.

4.2. Systemic corticosteroid therapy :

Two hundred and thirty-four patients (93%) received systemic corticosteroids (dexamethasone) at a mean dose of 8mg/day (4-

20mg/day).

4.3. Antibiotic therapy :

All patients received antibiotic therapy. The combination of a 3rd generation fluoroquinolone with a 3rd generation cephalosporin was the most prescribed (88.7%).

4.4. Anti-coagulant treatment :

Two hundred and thirty-three patients (93%) received preventive anticoagulant treatment. The remaining patients with pulmonary embolism or deep vein thrombosis received curative treatment.

4.5. Vitamin therapy :

All patients vitamin D3.

5. Evolution :

Progression was favourable in 79% of patients with improvement in their respiratory condition. Twenty-three patients (9.2%) presented with a worsening of their respiratory condition during hospitalisation.

A thoracic angioscan was performed in these patients, showing pulmonary embolism in five, lung abscess in two, pneumomediastinum in two and pneumothorax in one. Seven patients (3%) required transfer to intensive care with recourse mechanical ventilation. Death occurred in 21 patients (8.46%) as a result of respiratory distress.

DISCUSSION

The reference diagnostic method SARS-CoV2 infection is laboratory testing for viral RNA using RT-PCR (reverse transcriptase polymerase chain reaction) on nasopharyngeal swabs. However, it takes several hours to obtain the results, and only certain laboratories have this test. What's more, while the specificity of the viral test is excellent, its sensitivity is imperfect (60-70%) because it depends on the quality of the sample and the rate of viral replication in the upper respiratory tract [6-8]. Chest CT has rapidly established itself as an interesting diagnostic tool, given the often fairly characteristic presentation of COVID19 lesions [9]. In our study, thoracic CT was the main examination used to diagnose SARS-CoV2 infection, as it was requested in 99% of cases. The initial chest CT scan, performed without injection of contrast, is indicated in patients with dyspnoea and/or signs of acute respiratory failure, in order to ensure early therapeutic management and referral to COVID or non-COVID isolation units, in anticipation of RT-PCR results [10]. The sensitivity of CT scans for the diagnosis of COVID-19 is greater than 90%, with false negatives (normal scans when the disease is present) generally corresponding to patients who have been symptomatic for less than 3 days [8,11]. The specificity of CT scans varies. Chinese and Italian series have reported values of 25% and 56% respectively [8,12], but other series have reported values as high as 70%.In its COVID-19 imaging guidelines dated 11 June 2020, the WHO makes the following three recommendations for diagnosis [13]:

- In asymptomatic contacts of patients with COVID-19, the WHO suggests that imaging should not be used for diagnosis. An RT-PCR test should be carried out to confirm the diagnosis of COVID-19.
- In symptomatic patients with suspected COVID-19, the WHO suggests that chest imaging should not be used to diagnose COVID-19 when the RT-PCR test is available and results can be obtained rapidly.
- In symptomatic patients with suspected COVID-19, the WHO thoracic imaging to diagnose -COVID-19:

• the RT-PCR test is not available

• the RT-PCR test is available, but the results are slow in coming in

• the initial RT-PCR test is negative, but the clinical signs strongly suggest the presence of a COVID-19.

In our study, a thoracic CT scan was requested first, given the severe respiratory condition of our patients and the risk of delaying therapeutic management while awaiting the results of RT-PCR.

The most characteristic CT abnormalities in COVID-19 pneumonia are multifocal, bilateral, asymmetric ground-glass areas (about 80% of cases). Involvement classically predominates in the peripheral, posterior and basal regions [11,14,15]. There is generally no micronodular syndrome, excavation, septal lines or mediastinal adenomegaly. Other signs have been reported, such as the presence of fine reticulations, peribronchovascular thickening, peri- or intralesional vascular dilatations or signs of parenchymal distortion [15,16]. In our series, the radiological abnormalities detected by the thoracic CT scan were: ground-glass opacities (), bilateral involvement of the lesions, etc. (88%), peripheral distribution (43%), posterior topography of lesions () and parenchymal condensations (). Our results are similar those found in the two reviews of the literature by Salehi et al and Ye et al: ground-glass opacities (87%), bilateral involvement of lesions (80%), peripheral distribution (75%), multilobar involvement (89%), posterior topography of lesions (80%) and parenchymal condensations (33%) [15,17]. These ground-glass opacities have often been reported as being rounded, nodular or having a crazy-paving pattern. The lower lobes are the most affected and the middle lobe is the least affected by lung disease. Pure ground-glass opacities or opacities associated with condensations were one of the most frequently found patterns [14]. The frequency of these signs varies according to the studies and the stage of the disease. Other signs such as widening of vessels within frosted glass opacities, masses/nodules, halo or inverted halo signs, and linear opacities including thickening of the interlobular septa have been variably described [18].

In our series, pleural involvement was noted in 8% of cases. The presence of pleural effusion or pleural thickening isolated or adjacent to COVID-19 lesions has also been described [15, 17]. The meta-analysis by Bao et al [19], including 13 studies, showed that pleural fluid effusions were rarely observed (6%); they were rare in the initial phase of COVID-19 and occurred most often after the appearance of parenchymal opacities and often three weeks after the onset of pneumonia. In the systematic review by Ye et al [15], which included 14 studies of CT abnormalities in COVID-19, the prevalence of pleural effusions was 5%, ranging from 1% to 8%. In the work by Li et al [20], which included 83 patients, 25 of whom suffered from a severe form of COVID-19, pleural effusion was noted in 8.4% of cases (7/83), but only in severe forms (28%; n= 7/25). Pleural effusions appear to be rare COVID-19 (<10%). They are even rarer in the initial phase of the disease and most often occur 1 to 3 weeks after the appearance of parenchymal opacities. Another study [20] noted that pleural effusions were observed only in severe forms of COVID-19 (frequency of pleural effusions: 28%).

The imaging presentation of COVID-19 pneumonia varies according to the distinct stages of the disease, generally corresponding to phases of pneumonia organisation or diffuse alveolar lesions [21 ,22]. Some authors have proposed the following classification of stages of COVID-19 pneumonia according to the interval between symptom onset and chest CT: early phase, 0-5 days; intermediate phase, 6-11 days; and late phase, 12-17 days [22]. In fact, at the start of the disease (days 0-4 after the onset of symptoms), ground-glass opacities predominate and are located a limited number of lobes. As a reminder, more than half of patients may have a normal chest CT scan within the first 3 days. Over time, during the intermediate phase, we see the development of reticulations within the ground-glass areas ("crazy-paving"), but above all an extension of the lesions to include more lung segments and lobes. This is followed by appearance of condensations and mixed lesions (a combination of ground glass and condensations), some of which take on the characteristics of organised pneumonia (halo and inverted halo signs have been described, among others), and bands of curvilinear subpleural condensations considered by some to be typical of COVID-19 [23]. Reticulations associated with bronchiectasis and the development of irregular interlobular septal thickening have been observed after the second week of illness and suggest progression to fibrosis. CT findings coinciding with Clinical improvement shows a progressive resolution of the condensations, which give way once again to ground glass, and a regression in the number of lobes affected (also > D 14) [14, 24]. The maximum extent of parenchymal lesions occurs between 6 and 11 days (peak at D10) after the onset of symptoms and is consistent with the mean time of 10.5 days [25,26].

In our study, the involvement was atypical in 8% of cases. In almost 10 In some cases, the pulmonary involvement of COVID19 may be atypical and may take the form of pseudo-nodular condensations, sometimes accompanied by an inverted halo sign, suggesting a pattern of organised pneumonia.In our series, lung involvement was unilateral in 12% of cases. Unilateral presentations are possible in approximately 20-30% of cases, usually at an early stage before the lesions become bilateral [8,27]. Peribronchovascular or sometimes apical involvement has also been described [15,28]. When the infection occurs in a remodelled lung (e.g. emphysema, fibrosis), the classic peripheral multifocal presentation is rarely found, and comparison with previous examinations can be of great help. In order facilitate interpretation and improve communication of results between radiologists and clinicians, various societies and teams have emphasised the importance of structured and standardised reporting using clear and standardised radiological terms such as the CO-RADS (COVID-19 Reporting and Data System) and COVID-RADS classification systems [17,23]. The North American Radiology Society (RSNA) has proposed a 4-category classification of COVID-19 CT manifestations:

1) typical signs,

2) indeterminate, including less 'typical' symptoms,

3) Atypical: signs that have not been or are only exceptionally reported

4) negative with no sign of pneumopathy [29].

These classification systems would also have the advantage of increasing the specificity of imaging for the "typical" or "very high suspicion" categories of COVID-19 [23]. In the absence of, or pending, RT-PCR results, they must be interpreted in conjunction with clinical and biological data in order to clarify the clinical diagnosis of COVID-19.In addition, the French Society of Radiology has proposed a visual assessment of lesion extension, with several stages including minimal (<10%), moderate (10-25%), significant (26-50%), severe (51-75%) and critical (>75%) involvement. A greater risk unfavourable outcome has been observed in patients with significant and severe involvement on initial imaging [30]. Some studies support the predictive nature of this gradation of lesion extent on CT. Establishing lung damage scores would make it possible to assess the patient's prognosis and the need for intensive care unit management [16].In our seriesinvolvement was severe, with >50% involvement in 127 cases. (51%). During the initial assessment, there is no justification for systematically injecting scans. It is essential to know the date of onset of symptoms. Although thrombo-embolic complications are frequent in severe forms of the disease, generally from D10 onwards, the prevalence of pulmonary embolism during the first week does not appear to be higher than in a non-COVID population [31, 32]. However, there are two particular circumstances in which angioscan should be considered in the early phase:

-A discrepancy between absent or minimal pulmonary parenchymal lesions and a severe clinical picture compatible with PE.

-Very D-dimer levels.

There are no data validating a D-dimer threshold above which angioscan is indicated. Several publications suggest that the risk of pulmonary embolism becomes very high above a D-dimer threshold of 3000 μg/L [33,34].

In our series, a thoracic angioscan was requested immediately in 50 cases (20%). Pulmonary embolism was diagnosed in 19 patients (38%). Grillet et al [35] reported a positive rate of 23% for thoracic angioscan studies. In New York Kaminetzky et al [36] reported that when thoracic angioscan was performed, it was positive for PE in 37% of patients with COVID-19 compared with 14.5% of patients before the pandemic. A meta-analysis of 4,382 patients hospitalised with COVID-19 showed a 17.6% incidence of PE, with a significantly higher rate in patients with severe disease (21.7% vs. 12.5%) [37]. Thus, the incidence of PE varies considerably in the literature, and uncertainty remains as to who should have a thoracic angioscan [38].

In another multicentre study of 413 patients hospitalised with COVID-19 infection and suspected having pulmonary embolism (PE), PE was found in 25% of patients (95% CI: 21, 29).

Apart from clinical research protocols, there is no need to carry out a CT scan for therapeutic reassessment in clinically stable patients. In the event of a confirmed clinical deterioration, a thoracic angioscan is most often indicated. This examination is used search for pulmonary embolism. but also an adverse evolution in the form of ARDS, bacterial or aspergillary superinfection, or pneumothorax under mechanical ventilation [31].

Approximately 15-30% of patients hospitalised for SARS-CoV-2 infection progress to acute respiratory distress syndrome (ARDS), the leading cause of death in this population. ARDS is characterised on chest CT by bilateral parenchymal condensations predominantly in the declinal regions [5, 39].

In our series, 23 patients presented with a worsening of their respiratory condition during hospitalisation. A thoracic angioscan was performed in these patients, showing pulmonary embolism in five, lung abscess in 2, pneumomediastinum in two and pneumothorax in one. Several complications may also arise during the course of SARS-CoV-2 pneumonia. Bacterial superinfection of the lung parenchyma is suspected in the event of unilateral alveolar condensation associated with adenopathy and/or pleural effusions [16]. At present, there is no need to systematically inject CT scans performed as part of the initial work-up. However, if there is a clinical-radiological discrepancy (dyspnoea and hypoxaemia not explained by parenchymal abnormalities), the investigation should be continued with an injected CT scan. An injection is also advisable in the event of respiratory deterioration in a known COVID-19 patient, particularly in an intensive care unit. The value of injecting patients with very high D-dimer levels more systematically remains to be assessed.

CONCLUSION

Classified as a pandemic by the WHO on 11 March 2020, infection with COVID-19 (Corona Virus Disease 2019) represents a real medical challenge. Viral RNA testing by RT-PCR, the reference diagnostic technique until recently, has good specificity, but its sensitivity has been debated and was sometimes unavailable in certain centres during the first wave. Studies have therefore focused on demonstrating the value of performing a chest CT scan for diagnostic purposes. Certain CT lesions have been shown to be characteristic of COVID-19 infection. There is a temporal pattern to the appearance of the lesions described above, as well as a correlation between the extent of the lesions and the duration of the disease. If the diagnosis of COVID-19 pneumonia is suspected without any biological evidence, CT scans offer excellent diagnostic performance, with sensitivity of 90% and specificity of 91%. Chest CT therefore plays a key role in the management of COVID-19 pneumonia, particularly during the initial work-up, enabling rapid triage of dyspnoeic patients. In this context, we conducted a retrospective study including 251 patients admitted to the COVID-19 isolation unit between January and March 2021, 248 of whom (98.8%) had a chest CT scan on admission. The diagnosis of

SARS-COV2 infection was made on the basis of chest CT scans (in 119 patients: 48%) pending the results of RT-PCR, which was positive in 100 patients (84%). Only 112 patients (45%) were diagnosed on the basis chest CT. Chest CT combined with a positive rapid antigen test was used in 17 patients (7%). Chest CT without injection of iodinated contrast was performed in 198 patients (80%). A radiological appearance suggestive of COVID-19 pneumonia was found in 227 patients (92%); an atypical appearance of COVID-19 pneumonia was found in 21 cases (8%); abnormalities associated with typical COVID-19 pulmonary involvement were observed in 15% of patients. These included pulmonary embolism in 8% of cases and pleural effusion in 7%. in 8% of cases. Involvement was predominantly subpleural in 106 cases (43%), posterior in 87 cases (35%) and mixed in 108 cases. Lung involvement was bilateral in 217 cases (88%) and severe with an extent >50% in 127 cases (51%). The outcome was favourable in 79 of patients with an improvement in their respiratory condition. Twenty-three patients (9.2%) presented with a worsening of their respiratory condition during hospitalisation. A thoracic angioscan was performed in these patients, showing pulmonary embolism in five, lung abscess in two, pneumomediastinum in two and pneumothorax in one. The results of our study clearly show that chest CT is an essential tool for the positive diagnosis of COVID-19 pneumonia, particularly in patients with acute respiratory failure, either because of the unavailability of nasopharyngeal RT-PCR samples or the delay in obtaining the results of this test. Chest CT also plays an important role in the management of complications.

REFERENCES

1. Zhu N, Zhang D, Wang W, Li X, Yang B, Song J, et al. China Novel Coronavirus Investigating and Research Team.A Novel Coronavirus from Patients with Pneumonia in China, 2019. N Engl J Med. 2020 Feb 20;382(8):727-733. doi: 10.1056/NEJMoa2001017.

2. Kucharski AJ, Russell TW, Diamond C, Liu Y, Edmunds J, Funk S, et al. Early dynamics of transmission and control of COVID-19: a mathematical modelling study. Lancet Infect Dis 2020;20(5):553-8.

3. Wu Z, McGoogan JM. Characteristics of and Important Lessons From the Coronavirus Disease 2019 (COVID-19) Outbreak in China: Summary of a Report of 72,314 Cases From the Chinese Center for Disease Control and Prevention. JAMA. 2020 Apr 7;323(13):1239-1242. doi:10.1001/jama.2020.2648. PMID: 32091533.

4. Guan WJ, Ni ZY, Hu Y, Liang WH, Ou CQ, He JX, et al. China Medical Treatment Expert Group for Covid-19.Clinical Characteristics of Coronavirus Disease 2019 in China. N Engl J Med. 2020 Apr 30;382(18):1708-1720. doi: 10.1056/NEJMoa2002032. Epub 2020 Feb 28. PMID: 32109013; PMCID: PMC7092819.

5. Huang C, Wang Y, Li X, Ren L, Zhao J, Hu Y, et al. Clinical features of patients infected with 2019 novel coronavirus in Wuhan, China. Lancet. 2020 Feb 15;395(10223):497-506. doi: 10.1016/S0140-6736(20)30183-5. Epub 2020
Jan 24. Erratum in: Lancet. 2020 Jan 30;: PMID: 31986264; PMCID: PMC7159299.

6. Fang Y, Zhang H, Xie J, Lin M, Ying L, Pang P, et al. Sensitivity of Chest CT for COVID-19: Comparison to RT-PCR. Radiology 2020;19:200432.

7. Wang W, Xu Y, Gao R, Lu R, Han K, Wu G, et al. Detection of SARS-CoV-2 in Different Types of Clinical Specimens. JAMA. 2020 May 12;323(18):1843- 1844. doi: 10.1001/jama.2020.3786. PMID: 32159775; PMCID: PMC7066521.

8. Ai T, Yang Z, Hou H, Zhan C, Chen C, Lv W, et al. Correlation of Chest CT and RT-PCR Testing in Coronavirus Disease 2019 (COVID-19) in China: A Report of 1014 Cases. Radiology 2020;200642.

9. Pan F, Ye T, Sun P, Gui S, Liang B, Li L, et al. Time course of lung changes on Chest CT during recovery from 2019 novel Coronavirus (COVID-19) pneumonia. Radiology 2020;200370.

10. French High Council for Public Health. Avis du 23 mars 2020 relatif aux recommandations thérapeutiques dans la prise en charge du COVID-19 (complémentaire à l'avis du 5 mars 2020). Paris: HCSP; 2020.

11. Bernheim A, Mei X, Huang M, Yang Y, Fayad ZA, Zhang N, et al. Chest CT findings in Coronavirus disease-19 (COVID-19):relationship to duration of infection. Radiology 2020;200463.

12. Caruso D, Zerunian M, Polici M, Pucciarelli F, Polidori T, Rucci C, et al. Chest CT Features of COVID-19 in Rome, Italy. Radiology 2020;201237.

13. Akl EA, Blazié I, Yaacoub S, Frija G, Chou R, Appiah JA, et al. Use of Chest Imaging in the Diagnosis and Management of COVID-19: A WHO Rapid Advice Guide. Radiology. 2021 Feb;298(2):E63-E69. doi: 10.1148/radiol.2020203173.

14. Salehi S, Abedi A, Balakrishnan S, Gholamrezanezhad A. Coronavirus Disease 2019 (COVID-19): A Systematic Review of Imaging Findings in 919 Patients. AJR Am J Roentgenol. 2020 Mar 14:1-7. doi: 10.2214/AJR.20.23034.

15. Ye Z, Zhang Y, Wang Y, Huang Z, Song B. Chest CT manifestations of new coronavirus disease 2019 (COVID-19): a

pictorial review. EurRadiol. 2020 Aug;30(8):4381-4389. doi: 10.1007/s00330-020-06801-0.

16. Zhao W, Zhong Z, Xie X, Yu Q, Liu J. Relation Between Chest CT Findings and Clinical Conditions of Coronavirus Disease (COVID-19) Pneumonia: A Multicenter Study. AJR Am J Roentgenol. 2020 May;214(5):1072-1077.

17. Salehi S, Abedi A, Balakrishnan S, Gholamrezanezhad A. Coronavirus disease 2019 (COVID-19) imaging reporting and data system (COVID-RADS) and common lexicon: a proposal based on the imaging data of 37 studies. Eur Radiol. 2020 Sep;30(9):4930-4942.

18. Caruso D, Zerunian M, Polici M, Pucciarelli F, Polidori T, Rucci C, et al. Chest CT Features of COVID-19 in Rome, Italy. Radiology. 2020 Apr 3:201237. doi: 10.1148/radiol.2020201237.

19. Bao C, Liu X, Zhang H, et al. Coronavirus disease 2019 (COVID-19) CT findings: A systematic review and meta-analysis. J AmCollRadiol 2020;17:701-9.

20. Li K, Wu J, Wu F, Guo D, Chen L, Fang Z, et al. The Clinical and Chest CT Features Associated With Severe and Critical COVID-19 Pneumonia. Invest Radiol. 2020 Jun;55(6):327-331

21. Guan CS, Lv ZB, Yan S, Du YN, Chen H, Wei LG,et al . Imaging Features of Coronavirus disease 2019 (COVID-19): Evaluation on Thin-Section CT. AcadRadiol. 2020 May;27(5):609-613.

22. Li M, Lei P, Zeng B, Li Z, Yu P, Fan B, Wang C, Li Z, Zhou J, Hu S, Liu H. Coronavirus Disease (COVID-19): Spectrum of CT Findings and Temporal Progression of the Disease. AcadRadiol. 2020 May;27(5):603-608.

23. Prokop M, van Everdingen W, van Rees Vellinga T, Quarles van Ufford H, Stöger L, Beenen L, et al. COVID-19 Standardized Reporting Working Group of the Dutch Radiological Society. CO-RADS: A Categorical CT Assessment Scheme for Patients Suspected of Having COVID-19-Definition and Evaluation. Radiology. 2020 Aug;296(2):E97-E104.

24. Pan F, Ye T, Sun P, Gui S, Liang B, Li L, Zheng D, Wang J, Hesketh RL, Yang L, Zheng C. Time Course of Lung Changes at Chest CT during Recovery from Coronavirus Disease 2019 (COVID-19). Radiology. 2020 Jun;295(3):715- 721.

25. Wang Y, Dong C, Hu Y, Li C, Ren Q, Zhang X,et al . Temporal Changes of CT Findings in 90 Patients with COVID-19 Pneumonia: A Longitudinal Study. Radiology. 2020 Aug;296(2):E55-E64.

26. Shi H, Han X, Jiang N, Cao Y, Alwalid O, Gu J, et al. Radiological findings from 81 patients with COVID-19 pneumonia in Wuhan, China: a descriptive study. Lancet Infect Dis. 2020 Apr;20(4):425-434

27. Kanne JP. Chest CT Findings in 2019 Novel Coronavirus (2019-nCoV) Infections from Wuhan, China: Key Points for the Radiologist. Radiology 2020;295(1):16-7.

28. Chung M, Bernheim A, Mei X, Zhang N, Huang M, Zeng X, et al. CT Imaging Features of 2019 Novel Coronavirus (2019-nCoV). Radiology 2020;295(1):202-7

29. Simpson S, Kay FU, Abbara S, Bhalla S, Chung JH, Chung M, et al. Radiological Society of North America Expert Consensus Statement on Reporting Chest CT Findings Related to COVID-19. Endorsed by the Society of Thoracic Radiology, the American College of Radiology, and RSNA.J Thorac Imaging. 2020 Apr 28.

30. Leila Moulay Rchid. Prognostic value of chest computed tomography in patients hospitalized for COVID 19 pneumonitis. Life Sciences [q-bio]. 2020. ffdumas-03110659

31. Freund Y, Drogrey M, Miró Ò, Marra A, Féral-Pierssens AL, PenalozaA,et al. IMPROVING EMERGENCY CARE FHU

Collaborators. Association Between Pulmonary Embolism and COVID-19 in Emergency Department Patients Undergoing Computed Tomography Pulmonary Angiogram: The PEPCOV International Retrospective Study. AcadEmerg Med. 2020 Sep;27(9):811-820.

32. Jalaber C, Revel MP, Chassagnon G, Bajeux E, Lapotre T, Croisille P, et al Role of upfront CT pulmonary angiography at admission in COVID-19 patients.Thromb Res. 2020 Dec;196:138-140. doi: 10.1016/j.thromres.2020.08.037.

33. Tang N, Bai H, Chen X, Gong J, Li D, Sun Z. Anticoagulant treatment is associated with decreased mortality in severe coronavirus disease 2019 patients with coagulopathy. J ThrombHaemost. 2020 May;18(5):1094-1099.

34. Bompard F, Monnier H, Saab I, Tordjman M, Abdoul H, Fournier L,et al . Pulmonary embolism in patients with COVID-19 pneumonia. Eur Respir J. 2020 Jul 30;56(1):2001365.

35. Grillet F, Behr J, Calame P, Aubry S, Delabrousse E. Acute Pulmonary Embolism Associated with COVID-19 Pneumonia Detected with Pulmonary CT Angiography. Radiology. 2020 Sep;296(3):E186-E188.

36. Kaminetzky M, Moore W, Fansiwala K, Babb JS, Kaminetzky D,

HorwitzLI,et al. Pulmonary Embolism at CT Pulmonary Angiography in Patients with COVID-19. RadiolCardiothorac Imaging. 2020 Jul 2;2(4):e200308.

37. Liu Y, Cai J, Wang C, Jin J, Qu L. A systematic review and meta-analysis of incidence, prognosis, and laboratory indicators of venous thromboembolism in hospitalized patients with coronaviru disease 2019.J VascSurg Venous LymphatDisord. 2021 Sep;9(5):1099-1111.e6.

38. Ullah W, Saeed R, Sarwar U, Patel R, Fischman DL. COVID-19 Complicated by Acute Pulmonary Embolism and Right-Sided Heart Failure. JACC Case Rep. 2020 Jul 15;2(9):1379-1382.

39. Wang D, Hu B, Hu C, Zhu F, Liu X, Zhang J, et al. Clinical Characteristics of 138 Hospitalized Patients With 2019 Novel Coronavirus-Infected Pneumonia in Wuhan, China. JAMA. 2020 Mar 17;323(11):1061-1069.

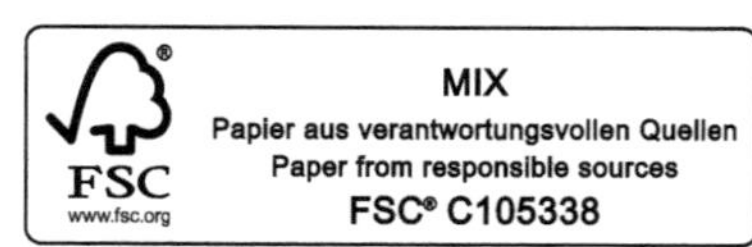

Printed by Books on Demand GmbH, Norderstedt / Germany